The Wonder

An Intersex Story

by Mac Del Ray

Produced by:

FriesenPress

Suite 300 – 852 Fort Street

Victoria, BC, Canada V8W 1H8

www.friesenpress.com

Distributed to the trade by The Ingram Book Company

Dedication

TO ALL INTERSEX INDIVIDUALS
IN THE WORLD TODAY

MAY YOU ALL ENJOY THE FREEDOM
AND THE WISDOM TO CHOOSE

Disclaimer

ALL NAMES CHARACTERS AND EVENTS
IN THIS STORY
ARE PURELY FICTITIOUS

RESEMBLANCE TO ANY EVENTS OR PERSONS
ALIVE OR DEAD
IS PURELY COINCIDENTAL
THE TITLE IS NOT BASED
ON ANY BOOK, IDEA OR
MOTION PICTURE

v I An Intersex Story

Foreword

Message to the Reader

In the spring of the year 2010, I returned from a pilgrimage in the South of India where I mainly visited holy sites in Andhra Pradesh and Tamil Nadu. Almost immediately, following my arrival back home, while I sat in front of my computer, a story began to unfold.

I had no idea where it was coming from as I had never had contact with Intersex persons in my life. Moreover, I had never heard or read the word Intersex.

Also, the title was born out of what had transpired at the end of the story and I had never heard of this word, wonder, used in any particular context other than when used in ordinary speech.

I came to the conclusion that something in this story needed to be shared with humanity at this time and that the information was required for its evolution.

Other than some basic editing, the story is basically unaltered from its original version.

Thank you for reading this story and for your interest in Intersex persons.

Mac del Ray

June 1st, 2013

I
A Special Birth

Henry was born with some very significant challenges. It was not unusual that he should sometimes feel lost and confused.

His mother was well intentioned. The truth was, she felt rather helpless herself, as to what to tell Henry and how to guide him. His father had not been able to cope with the reality of Henry when he was born; nor did he stay. One day, not long after she returned from the hospital, there was a note saying he was sorry but that he could not cope. He promised to send money on a regular basis.

When he came into the world, they could have made a choice for him but in truth, they were just too much in a state of shock to make any such decision so soon after the birth. They needed time to think, time to decide, time to react. They were numb.

Meanwhile, Henry was a jolly little fellow and a happier and more good-natured baby, there was none. Yet, they had no idea what the future held for someone like him...he might be condemned to secrecy all of his life.

Henry was born with both sets of sexual genitalia. For all intents and purposes, he was a complete hermaphrodite. They could have named him Sarah but they opted on a boy's name since the Doctor had said that his male genitalia seemed prominent. Chances are his hormones could be predominantly masculine and he could be more inclined to identify with his male side. There would be tests later on when he got older to determine exactly what was what.

Martha had to take a deep breath every time she changed or bathed him as she still had strong feelings regarding this kind of thing. Why did this have to happen to her? She was a very conservative woman who never asked for any trouble in her life. All she had ever wanted was an ordinary life with a husband and children. But now she only had a child. But, he was her flesh and blood and despite everything, she loved him.

She would have to plan everything out for him so that he would be protected from harm... so that those who did not love him the way that she did, would not judge him or want to punish or change him. She did not look forward to the time when he would turn twelve or thirteen. She thought about it and decided that he must be told sooner than that. She must make sure that he did not get the shock of his life when he discovered that no one else in their small town, was likely to be the way he was.

Martha thought best to tell him not long after he began grade school. For, as it turned out, nothing had been decided after Henry's birth. She had waited to see but nothing came of it. She let it slide. She could have decided to have her darling little boy's penis chopped off but she never had the heart to go through with it. She thought that God had made him this way and that, if later, he himself decided to have surgery, then, let it be his choice.

Her initial anxiety subsided and she began to realize how blessed she was. As he became a toddler and continued to grow, she loved Henry more every day and her heart became fuller and fuller with a love that she had not initially expected for this special little child.

Following her husband's departure, they still had a large light-filled house with front and back garden where Henry could play with the neighborhood children.

I I
The Dream

Henry had touched himself many times when he urinated and sometimes when he wanted to get to sleep. He knew he had some kind of a hole underneath his penis and ball sack but he thought everyone did. He seemed to be very normal as far as he was concerned.

He wondered why his mother was so uptight, when, as a toddler, he would run out of the toilet while forgetting to pull up his pants. She would always rush towards him and say, "No, no, Henry musn't do that!"... while quickly pulling them up.

Once, after a great day outside in the sunshine with his friends on the block, he came in ravenous. Martha had prepared a big dinner and he enjoyed every mouthful. She had even made his favorite, or at least, one of his favorite desserts, peach cobbler with butterscotch ice cream on top!

That night, after his bath, he didn't make a fuss to stay up for television despite the fact that it was summer holidays! He plopped right into bed and in no time, he was fast asleep. He had a deep, blissful sleep.

In the night, he went to a place where he had never been. His mother and he were in the car. She was silent but a heavenly music the likes that he'd never heard was playing on the radio. He was relaxing to the sound of this beautiful music coming in waves. The dream was in pink and violet shades.

They drove up a winding driveway to a magnificent building which reminded him of a castle much like what he might have seen in a book about a far off place in a fairy story. He opened the car door as he was anxious to stretch his legs. His mother stayed and said she would see him when he finished. He heard her comment but did not wonder what she meant.

He rang but since no one came to the door, he decided to let himself in. It was like a palace inside, all gold and jewels everywhere. A man appeared and greeted him; he said hello, and then when he looked again, he saw a woman; he was sure that a man had first appeared. Oh well, it didn't matter. The heavenly music continued as it did not seem confined to the car radio. He had never heard anything so beautiful in his entire life. He was curious to know what kind of instruments were playing.

The man/woman asked what he could he do for Henry. Henry replied that he had come for a visit. Next, he was ushered through a great long spacious corridor to a large hall where at the far end, he could see a man seated there on a sort of throne. The man who had showed him in announced him as "the young man" and he was told to come ahead.

Just as what had happened before, the seated man now appeared to be a woman. Henry was puzzled but somewhat amused. He did not have time to think about where this would lead to. The man said: "Good-day young man! Can I do something for you today?"

Henry said: "Good-day, Sir. Can you tell me how it is that you keep changing from a man to a woman then to a man again?" The wo/man replied: "In this country, everyone is this way; there is no difference between men and women; everybody is both. We are happy and complete this way and everyone is free to love anyone they are attracted to. We find that it is the best formula." Henry had no idea what to say, so he just replied: "Oh!"The wo/man then stated: "If you have any more questions, come back anytime."Henry, thinking that that was the best idea, turned around and said good-bye.

As he walked out through the long corridor, he realized that he was feeling very peaceful and that the wo/man's words had calmed him and made him feel an inner joy, a sort of quiet feeling, not the kind that would make him jump for it but a peaceful kind. He found his mother waiting as she said she would. They drove back in silence except that he could still hear that beautiful music and he was glad for it; he hoped that it would never stop.

When they arrived back home, his eyes opened and the music became a wonderful memory and he wondered if he would ever hear it again. He stayed in bed and mulled over the dream which was still fresh in his consciousness. He went over and over what the wo/man had said and he wondered what the relevance could be. He decided to keep it to himself and he remembered it from time to time.

He did not ascribe much more to it; after all, he was only six years old and it was another beautiful day and he needed to play with his friends again. They were waiting.

| | |
The Disclosure

That day was much like the day before. Henry had played and played totally spending all of his youthful energy. His mother had another great dinner prepared and another of his favorite desserts. That evening, something seemed different. She said, "Henry, after dinner, I want us to have a little talk." He replied, "Ok, mom."

So, they sat together in the living room and he could see that she was worried and anxious about something. He decided to say something: "What is it mom, what do you have to tell me?" She replied: "Son, you know I love you very much!"

"Of course, Mom! So, what is it?"

"There's something I've been meaning to tell you for some time but I wanted to wait until you were old enough to understand."

"Alright, Mom, what is it?" It seemed as though she would burst into tears at that moment, so he tried to reassure her, saying, "Mom, Mom, don't cry!"

Then, she took a very deep breath and started talking: "You know, Henry, how you have a penis down there...well, that's what boys have. And you know how, there 's a hole down there too. That's called a vagina. That's what girls have."

His reply, probably inspired by his recent dream was this: "I know, Mom, I know, and don't worry, it's alright!"

She was tearful and he hugged her and asked if he could watch a television program before bed. She said sure but to get ready for bed first. He scooted off and she wondered,

"What did all that mean?" He had taken it so well but surely he didn't really know what she had wanted to say to him. At least, the subject had been broached and she would discuss it again when she felt the time was right. Meanwhile, she thought, she should do a bit of research.

But, somehow, it wasn't until nearly two years later that she went to her computer and looked up hermaphroditism. She found the definition but learned that individuals who are Hermaphrodites, prefer the term Intersex as they feel that the former term is ambiguous and pejorative. She did some reading and was relieved to find that her instincts had been correct and that most intersex people resent surgery without their consent and prefer to decide for themselves.

Some time later, she found the courage to go back to the site. At the bottom of the page, she found a link to some support groups for intersex people and their families. She decided to look at the link.

IV
The Contact

Thinking back on her little talk with Henry, she realized just how fortunate she was in having such a wonderful child. A handsome blue eyed, blond boy, he was so joyful, with a purity and innocence in him that was hard to find in a human being. He was truly beautiful and sometimes she felt that he brought light into the room when he walked into it. Maybe that was what they meant when they spoke about spiritual people. In any case, she hoped that he never changed and that his present state of being would always shine through, whatever the future held. He seemed, to her, so full light and so insightful for such a small child.

She sat down at the computer again and wrote the following email:

"Dear Intersex Group"

She could not be more specific as she didn't know to whom she was writing. She guessed that there might be some secrecy involved in communicating with this type of group as one could never be sure who might be a kook or a crank trying to interfere in people's lives.

"I am the mother of Henry, an 8 1/2 year old Intersex child. I have been alone all my life with this secret and have recently begun to talk to my son about his condition. His father left soon after his birth as he said he could not cope with this. I feel that I have done right by Henry as I have not let the doctors alter him.

Now, though, I am in need of more support as Henry is growing up. Please let me know what kind of help there is for people like me and for Henry. Thank you very much."

She signed her first name only and sent it off. She waited patiently and the next day, there was a reply.

"Dear Martha"

Thank you for your enquiry. I am also a mother of an Intersex child. Like you, I struggle every day with the issues that lie before us. I have begun a support group for parents and later this will include a social group for the children. You are welcome to attend." She included her name and the time and place. It was in the next town that was only thirty minutes drive. She decided to attend once, just to see.

She had a babysitter come for Henry and drove off after lunch. It was not hard to find the address. When she rang, Marlene who had sent the email, answered the door and said, "Hello, you must be Martha, come in..."

Three other ladies were seated and they all introduced one another. Two of them said they had husbands who were at work and besides, they were too embarrassed to attend. She learned that the "group" had been formed not long ago and that they were feeling their way. The main thing they were looking for was support from one another. Marlene, the moderator noted: "It can get very lonely out there when you have something that you don't feel that you can discuss with anyone."

There was Carolyn who had Megan who is eight; Mary-Ann who has Benedict who is nearly ten and Lucy with Marvin who is also eight. Marlene has Taylor who is nine. Henry would soon be nine. So, they were all like her with the teenage years of their children coming up. They shared their stories and she also opened up about her Henry and how precious he was to her and how she wanted only what is best for him in every way. She stressed that she didn't want him hurt by the world!

There was coffee and they reconvened. Marlene said that she thought that it was time to start the social group. They talked about how that could be arranged. They decided that a Saturday activity could begin and they would see how that went and then, take it from there.

V
Dream States

That day was a very wet one, so wet that Henry had to come indoors and be babysat. That was not his favorite thing but when Agnes the lady who was babysitting him called him in, he did not make a fuss. He had his lunch and then, went to his room.

The rain had made him feel lethargic. He stretched out on the bed. No sooner had he closed his eyes, than that music, the music from the unusual dream he had had once came into his ears. He was transported back to the palace and in front of the wo/man once again. How strange! He was awake, yet "dreaming".

The wo/man greeted him once more and he noticed again that this person kept changing back and forth from being a man to a woman the way he had done on the first visit. He greeted Henry and asked how he was. Then, he asked if he wanted to have some friends?

As he began to speak, the whole scene vanished in front of his eyes, just as it had appeared and his eyes opened and he felt peaceful again, just as before.

It had been very short, this dream/vision. He was just going to say to the wo/man that he had friends but he didn't have the chancel! He wondered what that was all about! He did not regret that this had happened though, since it had left him feeling very relaxed and peaceful and he had heard the special music again. It had been a long time but he hadn't forgotten it!

VI
Friends

The next day, Martha asked Henry how he would like to come with her to meet some new "friends". He wasn't sure but he thought that she sounded a little mysterious; but he didn't have a problem with it. She said she had met some ladies and they would all get together with their children. It would be like a play date but with children his own age and the mothers would be there, at first. He said, "Sure, Mom."

So, off they went the following Saturday to meet the other mothers and the special children as she began to think of them. For a first meeting, Marlene had decided to host a barbecue. There were the five mothers from the first meeting and their five children. None of the husbands had chosen to attend. They weren't ready yet.

For some reason, Henry seemed to have made a connection between the "dream/vision" he had had and this meeting. He wasn't sure why but he was looking forward to this get together. He and his mother were last to arrive and he greeted everyone. He was pleased that the lady had a big back yard as he had brought his ball and mitt, hoping to play a bit. Benedict said he wasn't sure why they had all come to this barbecue as he had never heard his mother talk about any of these ladies before; Henry explained that a wo/man had asked if he had wanted to make some friends. No one thought twice about this comment but his mother thought why was he referring to her as a woman instead of as his mother.

Since Henry was so friendly and easy going, the other children decided to accept his invitation to play catch and they all formed a circle around the back garden while the mothers prepared the barbecue.

After awhile, it was time to eat and they all gathered round to the food area. They all piled food up on plates and took a lemonade and found a space out on the grass to have their own private picnic. All in all, it was a fun day and Henry seemed to enjoy his new friends. When it was time to leave, Henry said good-bye and in the car, he confided to his mother that he hoped that they would go back. She said she was glad that he had enjoyed it as she had agreed to host the next barbecue.

The following weeks they had get-togethers at each of the children's houses and they got to know one another; soon, some other children and mothers joined the group. The Mothers' Group also got together separately. At one meeting, they unanimously decided that it would be a good idea that all of the mothers should tell each of their children separately that all of the children in the friends' group were like them and that it was ok.

VII
All the Same

By this time, school had begun and Martha noticed that her boy was growing more and more handsome. Big for his age, he was certainly as mature as the others in the group. After dinner, one evening as he was doing his homework, Martha said that she would like to have a little chat later.

She invited him to have a snack before bed and she broached the subject. "Henry, I just wondered how you were doing in the friends' group we go to on Saturdays?"

He replied: "I like it fine, Mom; I really like the guys; they're cool. Why do you ask?"

"Well, I just wanted you to know something important about each and everyone of them. They are just like you. They are a little bit boy and they are a little bit girl and you know what, it's all ok."

"I know Mom, that it's ok, I mean. I had a dream about it once and the wo/man said that there are wo/men who are both men and women all at once. So, you know since then, if the wo/man says it's ok, then, it must be. Right, mom?"

"Right!"

"Good-night, Mom! I'm sleepy now...it's been a long day!"

VIII
Teenagers

Time elapsed and Henry continued to grow and mature. He did a lot of school work and he liked playing tennis after school. He enjoyed seeing Benedict and the other "special friends" as his mother called them, from the group. He looked forward to being with them all as he felt comfortable in the group. Since they were all, "the same", then, he knew that they could confide in one another when they felt the need to.

The mysterious dream-music which he loved so much, inspired him to learn to play the guitar; this took up much of his leisure time. He was becoming a sensitive and thoughtful young man and he even tried turning his thoughts and feelings into songs.

He was nearly fourteen and now it was summer again. He decided to invite Benedict to play tennis and for a visit. Tall and dark, he called himself Ben now that he was a teenager. Henry was happy to see his friend and glad that they had arranged for a sleep over. His Mom had gotten him a bunk bed for such occasions and he planned to let his friend have the top bunk since he was such a great guy!

After lights out, they talked. Ben said, "My mom says everybody in the "group" is like an angel since angels don't have one sex or the other."

Henry replied: "But we have both!" They laughed until their sides hurt!

The following week, at the "group", Megan started up by saying that she had something important to share. This was unusual. She was often outgoing and loud and today was no different.

"I have been going through some hard times, even if I always seem cheerful on the outside. I've been talking to a specialist doctor and I think I need to make a choice. I want to become a guy...only a guy."

Henry said: "Whatever you decide is fine Megan, we'll stand by you any way at all... "Everyone else, chimed in: "Yeah." Secretly, Henry thought that if she went through with it, then, really she could no longer belong to the "group". Each of the others wondered about that too but no one wanted to bring it up. It didn't seem to matter. In any case, things like that don't happen overnight; Megan could change her mind, who knows?

Days and months passed and many of the "group" members became seniors. One Saturday night, Megan called: "Hey Henry, I'm babysitting on Fairmont Avenue. Want to come over to help me babysit?" "Sure thing; just tell me the address; I can come for a bit but I have to be home by eleven."

So, there they were watching a movie and eating popcorn when, suddenly, Megan said, "Can I ask you a question, Henry?"

"Sure, go right ahead."

"Do you think I'm pretty?"

"Sure, Megan".

"I really like you Hen"...as she completed the statement, she moved over closer to where Henry was perched on the couch and kissed him.

"Megan, what do you think you're doing?"

"Why, Hen, didn't you like it?"

"Sure, Megan, but I just wasn't expecting it!"

"Hen, would you like it more if I were a boy? I was thinking about it before, remember?

"Yeah, but I don't know about that! Actually, I don't think it would make any difference. I guess, it's more of a personality thing!"

"What are you saying Henry, I don't have a good personality?"

"No Megan, that's not what I meant! It's just that sometimes people get along better with certain people. That's all!"

At that moment, he only just realized that there was one other person that he did like and that they were more suited to one another."

IX
Reunited

Ben was completing his first year in Pre-med at college and would be back for the summer. Henry would also be leaving at the end of the summer. Now, his thoughts were focused on Graduation.

He and Megan had decided to go together but not as a date; rather, since they were both graduating, they would just hang out together.

A few days before the Graduation, Henry had the dream again. This time, everything seemed in slow motion. His mother remained waiting in the car but a dark figure was also seated in the front seat. He did not see this person clearly. The palace was the same, golden and jeweled and he walked slowly down the long luxurious hallway.

When he arrived at the entrance to the Great Hall, the butler wo/man announced him.

"The young man has returned, your Excellency."

"Enter". "Welcome young Henry! Soon, you will embark on an important phase of your journey. Important people will return to you."

At that moment, he thought of Ben and how he looked forward to soon being reunited with his best friend. He stood there enjoying the wonderful heavenly music once again...then, the wo/man started fading and he returned to a conscious state.

X
Change

At the Prom, both Megan and Henry were happy to be together but they were feeling awkward just the same. They knew that many of the grads who were together tonight were amorous but they clearly were not and had never been inclined. As he drove her home she began confiding in Henry.

"I have come to a decision, Hen. I will see a surgeon and request the removal of my male genitals."

"Oh, Megan, are you sure?"

"Yes, Henry, I have been sure for a long time; I have just been waiting until I got older to go through with it. I don't feel that having male sexual features enhances my appeal in any way. If I could hope to have one of you love me, then, that would make it different. I need to love, so desperately."

"I'm sorry Megan, that I wasn't the one I could have been for you."

"Don't be Hen, you can't be attracted to someone as an obligation."

"So, what will you do?"

"My mom will take me to the city and we'll stay away all summer; that way, I'll recuperate before it is time to go away for school. It will just seem like I was away on a holiday."

"Oh, Megan!" said Henry as he gave his friend a big hug as they said "good-night."

XI
Important News

The next morning at breakfast, his mother brought up a subject that they rarely discussed.

"Henry, you know how you're always thinking out loud...I wonder what my Dad is like...well, your Dad, despite his having left us after you were born, has been providing for us all these years."

"Yes, Mom, I know that. You don't need to remind me."

"The reason I am reminding you Henry is that he called me yesterday."

"Really! What did he want?"

"Since you are turning eighteen, he wanted to know if he could see you. I told him I would leave it up to you to decide."

Henry's reaction was one of shock.

"I don't know Mom, can I think about it for a few days."

"Yes, dear, but don't wait too long; before long you'll be leaving for school!"

He went to his room and once again, thought about his recurring dream. Now, he knew who the dark unknown figure in the car must have been. And the wo/man had said that important people would be coming back into his life soon. Later, in the day, he told his mother that he agreed.

XII
A Realization

That night Ben and he got together. He had just returned from College that day and they couldn't wait to get together. When Ben arrived, they greeted one another warmly as they had not seen one another in months.

They felt that they had so much to catch up on. After dinner, with Martha out visiting a girlfriend, they had a chance to be alone. They sat in easy chairs in the living room.

Henry told Ben what was going on with Megan and he listened with great interest.

"She may have a point, you know, Hen! It can be very lonely out there for an ordinary straight person, let alone an Intersex one!"

"I felt that her decision could have been my fault. She said she liked me years ago and I couldn't like her back the way she would have wanted. I told her it wasn't personal but more a question of feeling comfortable."

"Hen, it's not your fault; Megan has to sort it our for herself. It is her life and her body. She is the only one who can decide."

"When I told her that, I realized for the first time, that there is someone else that I do feel more comfortable being with. "He looked at Ben and stared into his eyes for a long time in more than a friendly way. It did not take long for his friend to understand his meaning. Luckily, Ben had felt the same way for a very long time. He reached out and placed his hand in Henry's; they got up, embraced for a long time and walked arm in arm into the bedroom . When Martha returned, she locked the front door and switched off the house lights, having assumed that Henry and Ben were having a long-awaited sleep-over.

XIII
The Dark Stranger

Henry had asked Ben to accompany him to the city on the day that he was to meet his father for the first time. During the drive, Henry confided in Ben as he felt a growing intimacy between them. He shared a sense of Wonder which he said he had been aware of since he was born... a Wonder which was nurtured by his special dreams and the Dream-music which inspired him. He would be studying Music Composition in the fall at University. He hoped that they could share a flat together. Ben seemed to be on the same wavelength and said that he had also thought about being with Henry.

The Wonder also applied to the Intersex part of them. Henry shared with Ben how life was so special and how God had made them very unique to be able to love anyone of their choice. He felt that Ben was particularly suited to him as he was to Ben and each of them complemented the other in their own very distinctive way. He felt that this was very unusual and that in the world, they would have a difficult if not impossible task of ever finding anyone else who could be what they were to one another.

He had asked Ben to come with him for support but he wanted him to wait outside while he went up to his father's office. He felt anxious to meet this man who was finally showing a genuine interest in him.

Ben parked, giving Henry's hand a firm squeeze and warmly saying: "I'll meet you out front in one hour." Henry went up to the seventh floor and found the door with the name of the Company that his father worked for. Cautiously, he opened the door and stepped in.

At the front desk, he asked for Mr. Patten. He was told to take a seat and not long after, he was shown the way down the corridor into his father's office.

He opened the door and found a man seated at a large desk which was framed by a wall of windows. The man who was his father stood up and held out his hand for a shake. Henry shook it and sat down when invited to do so.

His father began:

"Henry, I'm sorry that I have been absent from your life for all of these years."

At that moment, his father's words brought to his consciousness a torrent of built-up emotion and he started sobbing.

"Please forgive me, son."

Coming around from the desk, his father sat beside Henry and put his arm around him.

An hour later, Ben was outside waiting for his friend. Henry came out a few minutes later, looking mysterious and pleased. They hugged in a warm embrace. The Wonder appeared to have taken over once again.

The End